CBB

Nursing Assessment of the Neurological Patient

Written and Published by
Claudia Barros MSN RN CCRN
7821 North 173rd Avenue
Waddell AZ 85355

Do not duplicate, disseminate, or appropriate this book without written permission of the author.

About the Author

Claudia Barros is a Masters prepared Registered Nurse with over 25 years critical care practice.

She has practiced in various critical care settings including CCU, CVICU, Surgical ICU, Medical ICU, Transplant, Trauma and Post Anesthesia Care.

Claudia has taught nursing in both the clinical and classroom setting.

She has developed curriculum for the 3rd and 4th semesters of nursing, designed and implemented a Paramedic to RN program, and created Simulation scenarios for all of her courses at the college level.

Chapters

Chapter 1 .... page 5
Introduction to the Neurological Assessment

Chapter 2 .... page 9
Assessing Pupillary Function
Pupillary Size Chart in Millimeters

Chapter 3 .... page 11
Utilizing the Glascow Coma Scale

Chapter 4 .... page 13
Categories of Consciousness
Assessing the Unconscious Patient

Chapter 5 .... page 14
Assessing Muscular Strength
Testing Upper Body Strength
Testing Lower Body Strength
Muscle Strength Scale
Classification of Abnormal Motor Function

Chapter 6 .... page 17
The Cranial Nerves Assessment
The Six Cardinal Fields of Gaze

Chapter 7 .... page 26
The Babinski Reflex

Chapter 8 .... page 27
The Dermatomes
Assessing the Dermatomes

Chapter 9 .... page 30
Post Anesthesia Care Unit Assessment
The Aldrete Score

Chapter 10 .... page 33
Administering Sedation
MAAS, RASS and CAM-ICU Assessments

Chapter 11 .... page 38
NIH Stroke Scale Assessment

Chapter 12 .... page 41
Neurological Patient Case Studies
Sedation and Epidural Anesthesia Questions

In Summary .... page 60

Chapter 1

Introduction to the Neurological Assessment

A neurological examination is the assessment of consciousness, sensory responses and motor functions, including reflexes, to determine whether the nervous system is impaired.

The neurologic examination typically includes a physical examination and a review of the patient's medical history. The examination can be used as a screening or investigative tool to determine if there are neurological deficits or abnormalities.

A neurological examination is ordered when a physician suspects a patient may have a neurological disorder or when the patient is neurologically impaired due to illness, injury, surgical interventions or from the effects of sedation and analgesics.

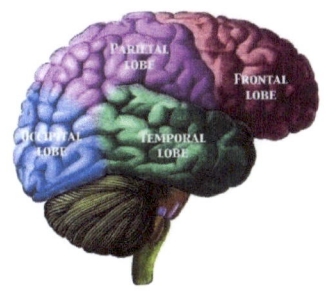

Patient History

The patient's history is an important part of a neurological examination. Factors to be considered in the medical history include:
- Time of onset, duration and associated symptoms
- Age, gender, and occupation
- Handedness
- Past medical history
- Drug history
- Family and social history

Neurological Tests

Specific tests used in a neurological examination include:
- Pupillary Response
- Glasgow Coma Scale
- Level of Consciousness
- Motor Function Evaluations
- Cranial Nerves Assessment
- Deep Tendon Reflexes
- Sensory Nerve Evaluations
- Assessments related to Anesthesia, Sedation, Paralytics and Analgesics
- Stroke Evaluation

General Principles of the Neurological Examination

Testing neurological function and integrity can easily be incorporated into the nurse's daily routine. Talking with a patient can help the nurse assess orientation and level of consciousness. Asking the patient to perform simple tasks, such as reaching and grasping can evaluate motor function.

The central nervous system (CNS) includes the brain and spinal cord. CNS assessments will allow the nurse to evaluate patients post-operatively, patients suspected of having a stroke or head injury, and patients receiving sedation.

The peripheral nervous system includes the peripheral and cranial nerves. The nurse can assess motor function, reflexes and sensory deficits either from injury or anesthetics.

The Neurological Assessment

The following chapters explain how to perform each component of the neurological assessment. How often each assessment must be completed is based upon the physician orders and the patient's condition.

Typically, the nurse will complete each component of the neurological assessment every 1 to 4 hours. The nurse can use his or her judgement to increase the assessment frequency when the patient's condition worsens.

In order to perform the neurological assessment less frequently, the nurse will need to obtain a physician order specifying the neurological assessment frequency.

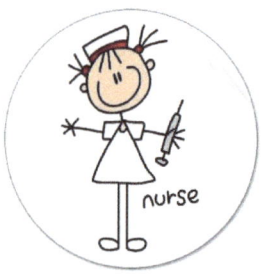

Chapter 2

Assessing Pupillary Function

Nursing priorities should focus on:

- Estimating pupil size and shape
    - In millimeters
    - Regular or irregular
- Evaluating each pupil's reaction to light
    - Brisk or Sluggish
    - Fixed or Dilated
- Assessing eye movement (dolls eyes)
- To assess dolls eyes
    - Hold eyes open and turn patient's head briskly to side, if the eyes deviate to the opposite side the oculocephalic reflex is intact.
    - If the eyes remain midline or move with the head, this indicates significant brain stem injury.
- Pupillary function should be assessed and documented every 1 to 4 hours as a part of the neurological and physical assessment.

Pupillary Size Chart in Millimeters

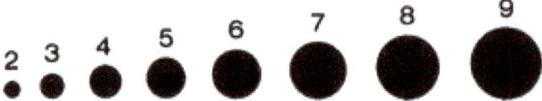

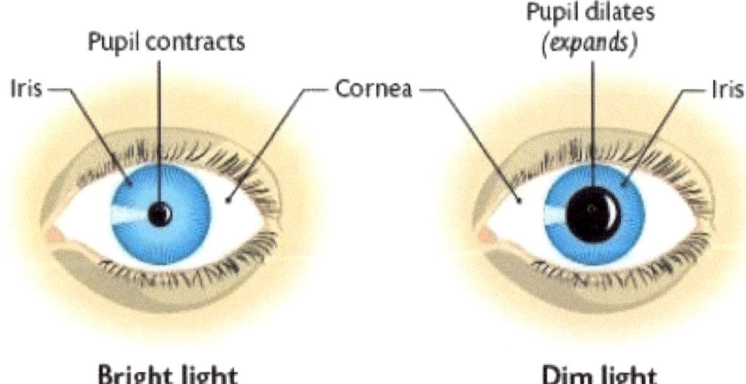

Bright light   Dim light

Chapter 3

Utilizing the Glascow Coma Scale

- The Glascow Coma Scale (GCS) is a standardized scale used to evaluate neurological response.
- The scale is divided into three sections designed to assess consciousness, verbal abilities, and motor response.
- The score ranges from 3 to 15 with 15 representing normal function.
- The scale is a useful tool to assess and communicate the patient's neurological condition, including any deficits or signs of increased intracranial pressure.
- The Glascow Coma Scale should be assessed and documented every 1 to 4 hours as part of the neurological and physical assessments.

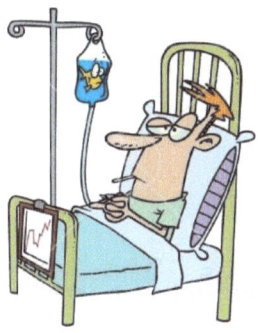

GLASCOW COMA SCALE	SCORE
Best Eye Opening Response	
• Spontaneous	4
• To Speech	3
• To Pain	2
• None	1
Best Motor Response	
• Obeys Commands	6
• Localizes Pain	5
• Flexion Withdraw to Pain	4
• Decorticate	3
• Decerebrate	2
• No Movement	1
Best Verbal Response	
• Oriented Conversation	5
• Confused Conversation	4
• Inappropriate Words	3
• Incomprehensible Sounds	2
• No Vocalization	1

Chapter 4

Categories of Consciousness

Consciousness is assessed and documented every 1 to 4 hours as part of the neurological and physical assessments.

Alert	Patient responds immediately to minimal external stimuli.
Confused	Patient is disoriented to time or place but usually oriented to person, with impaired judgment and decision making and decreased attention span.
Delirious	Patient is disoriented to time, place, and person with loss of contact with reality and often has auditory or visual hallucinations.
Lethargic	Patient displays a state of drowsiness or inaction in which the patient needs an increased stimulus to be awakened.
Obtunded	Patient displays dull indifference to external stimuli, and response is minimally maintained. Questions are answered with a minimal response.
Stuporous	Patient can be aroused only by vigorous and continuous external stimuli. Motor response is often withdrawal or localizing to stimulus.
Comatose	Vigorous stimulation fails to produce any voluntary neural response.

Assessing the Unconscious Patient

- First, try to stimulate a response verbally, in a soft tone.
- Second shout "Wake up."
- Third, shake patient firmly.
- Fourth, illicit a response by using painful stimuli such as trapezius squeeze, supraorbital, mandibular or nail bed pressure, or sternal rub.

Chapter 5

Assessing Muscular Strength

- This part of the neurological assessment can help identify motor weakness.
- When testing strength allow for variability due to age, sex and physical fitness.
- Remember the dominant side is usually slightly stronger.

Testing Upper Body Strength

- Test flexion and extension at the elbow by having the patient pull and push against your hand.
- Test grip strength by asking patient to squeeze two of your fingers as hard as possible and to not let go as you pull away.
- Test extension at the wrist by having the patient make a fist and resist you from pulling it down.

Testing Lower Body Strength

- Test flexion of the hip by placing your hand on the patient's thigh and asking them to raise their leg upward against your hand.
- Test extension at the knee by supporting the knee in flexion and asking the patient to straighten their leg against your hand.
- Test flexion at the knee by placing the patient's leg so the knee is flexed with the foot resting on the bed. Have the patient keep their foot down while you attempt to straighten their leg.
- Test dorsiflexion and plantar flexion at the ankle by asking the patient to pull up, then push down against your hand.
- Muscle strength is assessed and documented every 1 to 4 hours as part of the neurological and physical assessments.

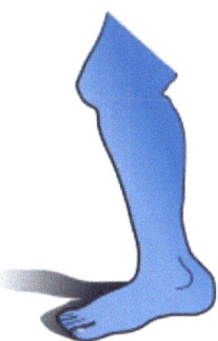

Muscle Strength Scale

0	No muscular contraction
1	Barely detectable flick
2	Active movement with gravity eliminated
3	Active movement against gravity
4	Active movement against gravity & some resistance
5	Active movement against full resistance without evidence of fatigue. Normal strength.

Classification of Abnormal Motor Function

Spontaneous	Occurs without regard to external stimuli and may not occur by request
Localization	Occurs when the extremity opposite the extremity receiving pain crosses midline of the body in an attempt to remove the noxious stimulus from the affected limb
Withdrawal	Occurs when the extremity receiving the painful stimulus flexes normally in an attempt to avoid the noxious stimulus
Decortication	Abnormal flexion response that may occur spontaneously or in response to noxious stimuli
Decerebration	Abnormal extension response that may occur spontaneously or in response to noxious stimuli
Flaccid	No response to painful stimuli

Chapter 6

The Cranial Nerves Assessment

Picture This!

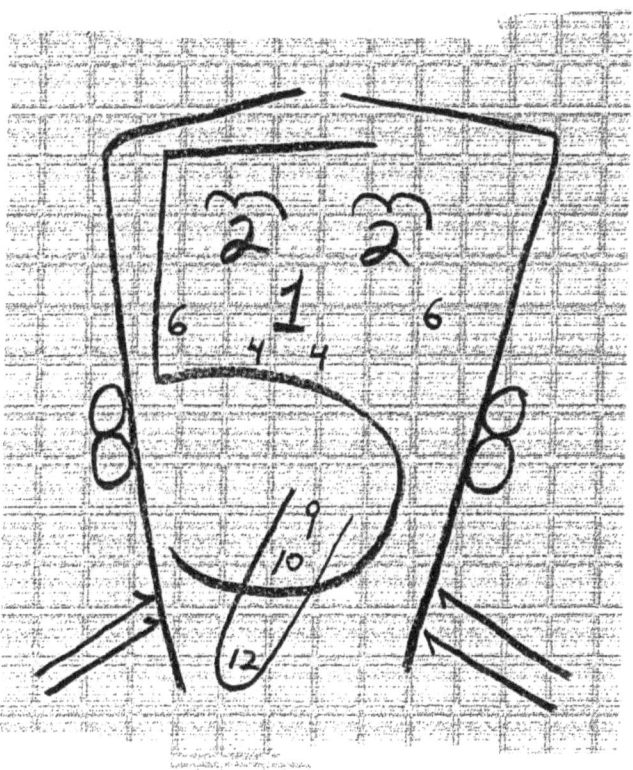

The cranial Nerves should be assessed and documented every 1 to 4 hours as part of the neurological and physical assessments.

Olfactory nerve (CN I)

- Located in the nose, cranial nerve CN I controls the sense of smell. This nerve is not frequently tested, even by neurologists. However, suspect an abnormality in this nerve when a neurologic patient has a poor appetite.
- To assess the nerve, use soap or coffee — both can easily be found on the nursing unit. Do not use a substance with a harsh odor, such as ammonia, because it will stimulate the intranasal pain endings of CN V.
- Have the patient close both eyes, close one nostril, and gently inhale to smell the scent. Remember to test both nostrils.

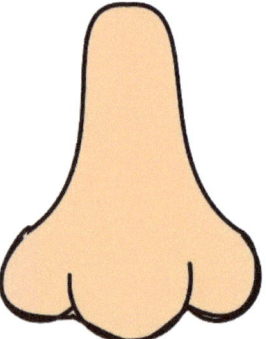

Optic nerve (CN II)

- Located in and behind the eyes, CN II controls central and peripheral vision.
- The fovea in the center of the retina is responsible for visual acuity in the central vision. Test one eye at a time. Ask the patient to read their I.V. bag. Then have the patient count how many fingers you are holding up 6 inches in front of him or her.
- Test peripheral vision one eye at a time. Cover one of the patient's eyes and instruct the patient to look at your nose. In the patient's superior (upper) and inferior (lower) peripheral fields of vision wiggle your index finger. Ask the patient to note any movement in the peripheral visual fields as you wiggle your finger.

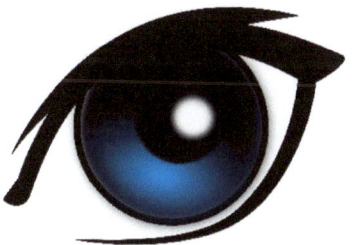

Oculomotor nerve (CN III)

- Also positioned in and behind the eyes, CN III controls pupillary constriction.
- To test the patient's pupils, dim the lights, bring the light of the penlight from the outside periphery to the center of each eye, and note the response. Use the mm chart to describe pupil size; descriptions such as "small," "medium," and "large" are too subjective.
- Also, check where the eyelid falls on the pupil. If it droops, note that the patient has ptosis.
- It is easy to check cranial nerves III, IV, and VI together.

Trochlear nerve (CN IV)

- Cranial nerve IV acts as a pulley to move the eyes down — toward the tip of the nose.
- To assess the trochlear nerve, hold your index finger approximately 12 inches in front of the patient's nose then instruct the patient to follow your finger. Slowly move your finger towards their nose and observe for normal crossing of the eyes.

Trigeminal nerve (CN V)

- Cranial nerve V covers most of the face.
- If a patient has a problem with this nerve, it usually involves the forehead, cheek, or jaw — the three areas of the trigeminal nerve. Check sensation in all three areas, using a soft and dull object. Check sensation of the scalp, too.
- Test the motor functions of the temporal and masseter muscles by assessing jaw opening strength. If you suspect a problem with cranial nerves VI and VII, check the corneal reflex with a cotton wisp since it is easy to do this while you are checking trigeminal nerve function.

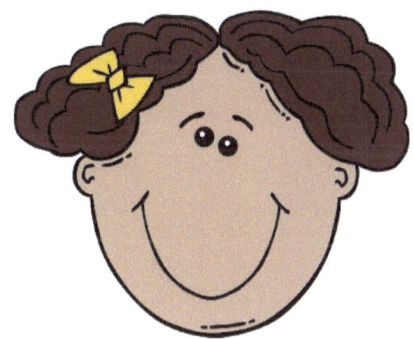

Abducens nerve (CN VI)

- Cranial nerve VI controls eye movement to the sides.
- Ask the patient to look toward their right ear. Then have the patient follow your index finger through the six cardinal fields of gaze.
- With your index finger, draw a big X in the air and then draw a horizontal line across it.
- Observe the patient for nystagmus or twitching of the eye.

Six Cardinal Fields of Gaze

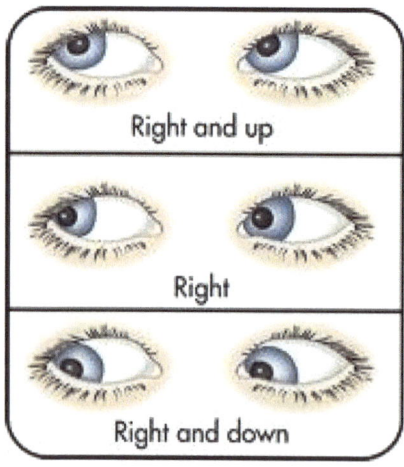
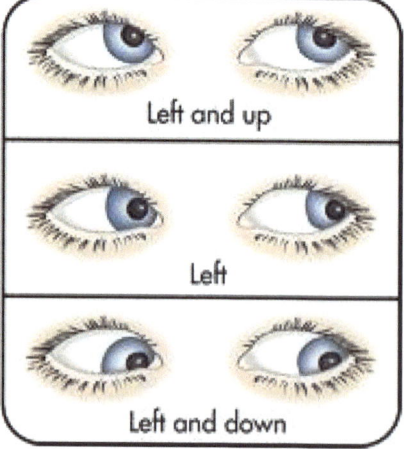

Facial nerve (CN VII)

- Cranial nerve VII controls facial movements and expression.
- Assess the patient for facial symmetry.
- Have the patient wrinkle their forehead, close their eyes, smile, pucker their lips (like a kiss), show their teeth, and puff out their cheeks. Both sides of their face should move symmetrically.
- When the patient smiles, observe the nasolabial folds (smile lines) for weakness or flattening.

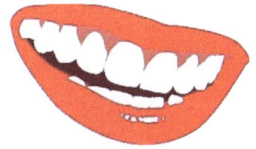

Acoustic nerve (CN VIII)

- Cranial nerve VIII, located in the ears, controls hearing.
- Check hearing by rubbing your fingers together by each ear.

Glossopharyngeal nerve (CN IX) and Vagus nerve (CN X)

- Cranial nerves IX and X, which innervate the tongue and throat (pharynx and larynx), are checked together.
- Assess the sense of taste on the back of the tongue.
- Observe the patient's ability to swallow by noting how he or she handles secretions.
- Ask the patient to open their mouth and say *AHHHHHH*.
- The uvula should be in the midline, and the palate should rise.

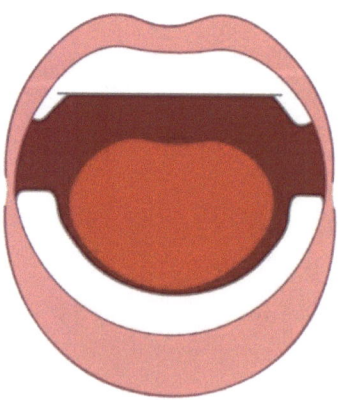

Spinal accessory nerve (CN XI)

- This nerve controls neck and shoulder movement.
- Ask the patient to raise their shoulders against your hands to assess the trapezius muscle.
- Then ask the patient to turn their head against your hand to assess the sternocleidomastoid muscle.

Hypoglossal nerve (CN XII)

- Cranial nerve XII innervates the tongue.
- Ask the patient to stick out their tongue. It should be in the midline.
- Look for problems with eating, swallowing, and speaking.
- You can check this nerve when you check cranial nerves IX and X.

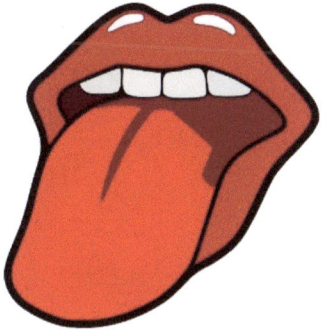

Chapter 7

The Babinski Reflex

- The lateral side (outer aspect) of the sole of the foot is rubbed with a blunt implement so as not to cause pain, discomfort or injury to the skin.
- The blunt instrument is run from the heel along a curve to the toes.
- The Babinski reflex should be assessed and documented every 1 to 4 hours as part of the neurological and physical assessments.

- Negative Babinski - the toes curve inward. This is the response seen in healthy adults.

- Positive Babinski - the toes fan out. This response indicates damage to the Central Nervous System.

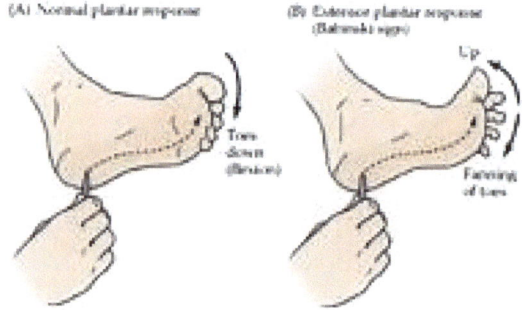

Chapter 8

The Dermatomes

- The human body can be divided into regions that supply specific areas of the skin with sensation. These regions each arise from a single spinal nerve and are known as Dermatomic Areas or Dermatomes.
- The spinal nerves which form the dermatomes include eight cervical (one for the head and one for each cervical vertebrae), twelve thoracic, five lumbar and five sacral.
- These spinal nerves innervate the body in a patterned form. Along the thorax and abdomen, the dermatomes are stacked like discs forming a human torso, each supplied by a different spinal nerve.
- Along the arms and legs, the pattern is different: the dermatomes run longitudinally along the limbs.
- Dermatomes are useful in neurology for finding the site of spinal cord injury and in anesthesia for assessing the level of epidural anesthesia (spinal block).

Assessing the Dermatomes

Assessing the level of injury or epidural anesthesia is easy and quick.

The nurse will need:
- An alcohol wipe or ice cube to assess the sensation of cold.
- A sharp needle or pin.
- Assess the patient first on an area of skin where the nurse knows the patient has normal sensation.
- Then assess above and below the area of injury or anesthesia.
- Do not forget to assess both the right and left side.
- Document the level of normal sensation based upon the Dermatome chart.
- The dermatomes are assessed along with vital signs, pain, sedation and level of consciousness every 15 minutes for 1 hour, then every hour for 24 hours, and then every 4 hours.

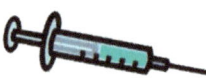

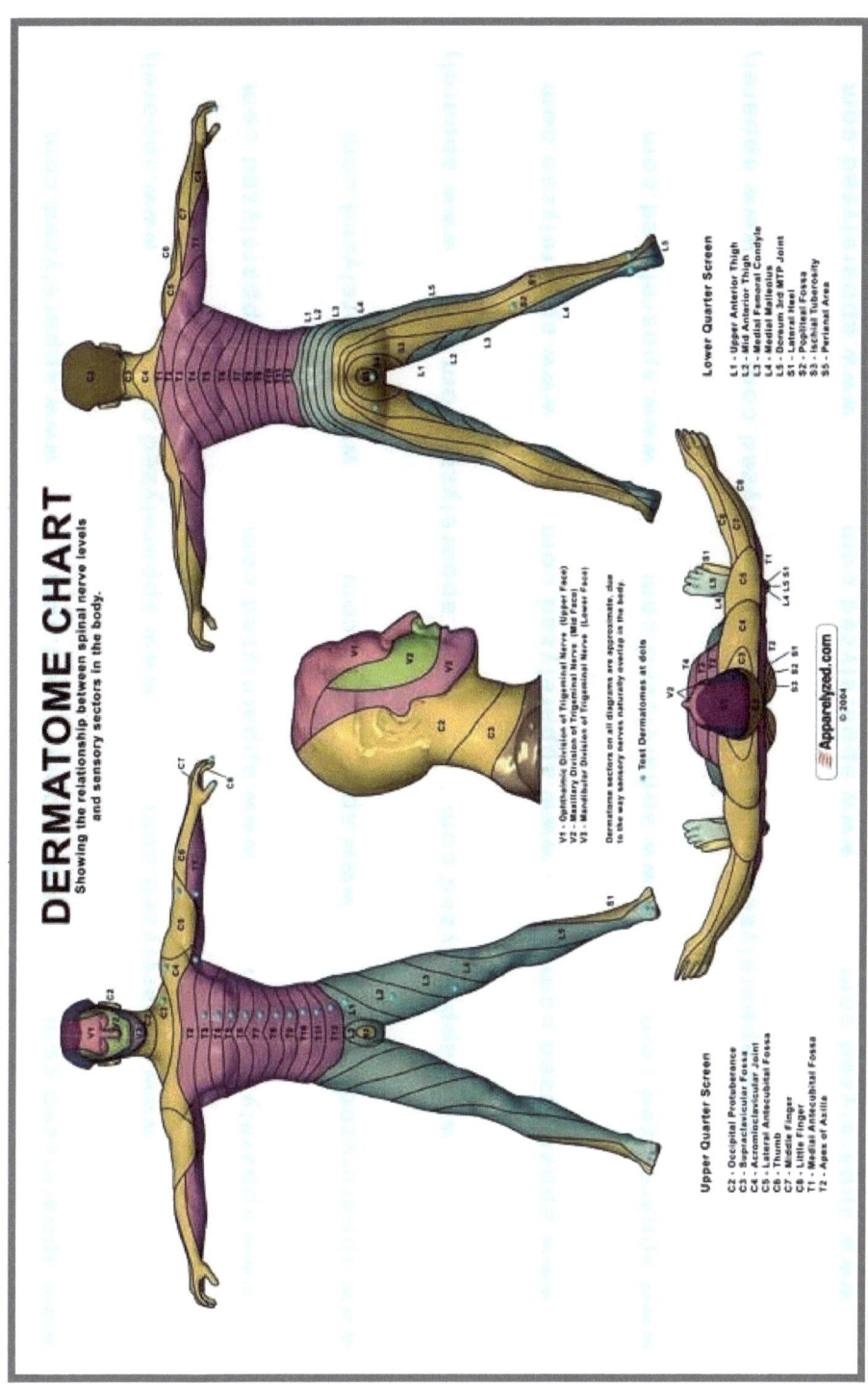

Neurological Assessment

Chapter 9

Post Anesthesia Care Unit (PACU) Assessment

- The Aldrete Score is used by nurses in PACU during the post-operative period to evaluate a patient's recovery from anesthesia.
- The patient is assessed and scored based upon motor activity, respiratory status, circulatory status, level of consciousness, and skin color.
- The nurse assigns a score of 0 through 2 for each category with a maximum score of 10.
- The Aldrete score is used as a criteria for discharge from the PACU.
- The Aldrete score can also be used to assess the patient during and after procedural sedation.

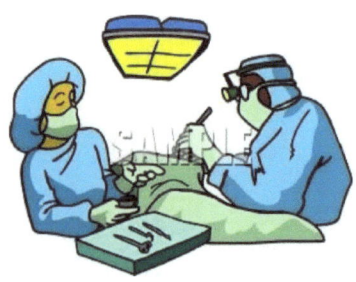

Practice Standards when using the Aldrete Score

- The standard of practice for use of the Aldrete Score is established by the American Society of PeriAnesthesia Nurses (ASPAN).
- The routine assessment and documentation of the Aldrete score post-operatively includes vital signs and pain assessment.

- The score should be calculated every 5 minutes times 3, every 15 minutes times 4, every 30 minutes times 2, and then every hour until the patient achieves a score that matches or exceeds their pre-anesthesia or pre-procedural sedation score.
- If a patient's score is 8 or below, the anesthesiologist must be notified and the patient cannot be discharged from the PACU or discharged home post procedure.

The Aldrete Score

ALDRETE - Post Anesthesia Score	
ACTIVITY	Able to move 4 extremities voluntarily or on commands = 2 Able to move 2 extremities voluntarily or on commands = 1 Able to move 0 extremities voluntarily or on commands = 0
RESPIRATIONS	Able to deep breath and cough freely = 2 Dyspnea or limited breathing = 1 Apneic = 0
CIRCULATION	BP +/- 20% preanesthesia level = 2 BP +/- 20-50% preanesthesia level = 1 BP +/- 50% preanesthesia level = 0
CONSCIOUSNESS	Fully awake = 2 Arousable on calling = 1 Not responding = 0
COLOR	Pink = 2 Pale, dusky, blotchy, jaundiced = 1 Cyanotic = 0

Chapter 10

Administering Sedation

- Adequate sedation or paralytics (intermittent or continuous) should be used to prevent movement and coughing during suctioning in order to decrease intracranial pressure, control temperature, and promote hemodynamic stability.
- When a neuromuscular block is used, continuous sedation must be employed. Short-acting drugs, such as Propofol or Precidex, may be used.
- Concurrent analgesia should always be considered when neuromuscular blocks and / or sedation agents are administered. Morphine and fentanyl are frequently used in conjunction with sedation and paralytics in ventilated intensive care patients.

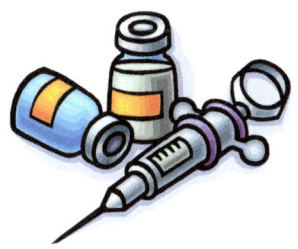

- The use of sedation agents, paralytics and analgesics will interfere with the ability to perform a proper neurologic examination.
- Use minimal sedation and analgesics to allow for accurate neurological assessments.
- The titration of any specific agent should be tailored to the desired level of sedation.
- There should always be an assessment of the level of sedation and whether it is effective.
- Level of sedation can be assessed subjectively through clinical examination or objectively with the use of tools such as MAAS, RASS or CAM-ICU.
- Assessment of the patient's level of pain should also be completed and documented when administering analgesic agents.
- Monitor sedation level and pain assessment every 1 to 4 hours depending on the patient's clinical findings.

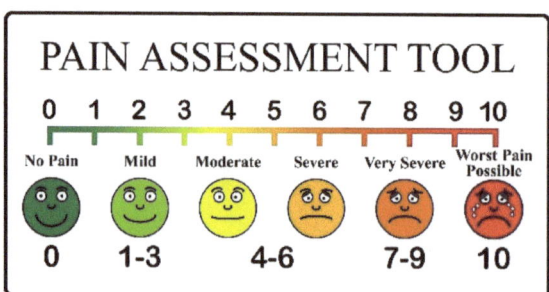

Neurological Assessment

Motor Activity Assessment Scale (MAAS)

SCORE	DESCRIPTION
0	Unresponsive to noxious stimuli.
1	Responsive (opens eyes, raises eyebrows, turns head, moves limbs) with noxious stimuli.
2	Responsive (opens eyes, raises eyebrows, turns head, moves limbs) to touch or when name loudly spoken.
3	Calm and cooperative (No external stimuli required to elicit movement AND patient is purposeful and follows commands).
4	Restless and cooperative (No external stimuli required to elicit movement AND patient is uncovering self or picking at sheets or tubes).
5	Agitated (Consistently does not follow commands, attempts to sit up or climb out of bed).
6	Dangerously agitated / uncooperative (e.g. patient is thrashing, pulling at tubes, striking at staff, climbing out of bed, not calming down when asked).

Noxious Stimuli: Suctioning or 5 seconds of vigorous orbital, sternal, or nail bed pressure.

Richmond Agitation-Sedation Scale (RASS)

Sedation Assessment

Score	Label	Description
+4	Combative	Overtly combative, violent, immediate danger to staff
+3	Very Agitated	Pulls or removes tubes or catheters; aggressive
+2	Agitated	Frequent non-purposeful movement, fights ventilator
+1	Restless	Anxious but movement not aggressive, vigorous
0	Alert and Calm	
-1	Drowsy	Not fully alert but has periods of sustained awakening; Eye-opening or eye contact to voice for greater than 10 seconds
-2	Light Sedation	Briefly awakens to voice with eye contact for less than 10 seconds
-3	Moderate Sedation	Movement or eye opening to voice but no eye contact
-4	Deep Sedation	No response to voice, but movement or eye opening to physical stimulation
-5	Unarousable	No response to voice or physical stimulation

If RASS is greater than or equal to -3 complete the CAM-ICU Assessment

If RASS is -4 or -5 STOP (patient unconscious) RECHECK later

Confusion Assessment Method for the Intensive Care Unit (CAM-ICU)

Confusion Assessment Method for the ICU (CAM-ICU) Flowsheet

1. Acute Change or Fluctuating Course of Mental Status:
- Is there an acute change from mental status baseline? OR
- Has the patient's mental status fluctuated during the past 24 hours?

→ NO → **CAM-ICU negative NO DELIRIUM**

→ YES ↓

2. Inattention:
- "Squeeze my hand when I say the letter 'A'."
Read the following sequence of letters: S A V E A H A A R T
ERRORS: No squeeze with 'A' & Squeeze on letter other than 'A'
- If unable to complete Letters → Pictures

→ 0-2 Errors → **CAM-ICU negative NO DELIRIUM**

→ > 2 Errors ↓

3. Altered Level of Consciousness
Current RASS level

→ RASS other than zero → **CAM-ICU positive DELIRIUM Present**

→ RASS = zero ↓

4. Disorganized Thinking:
1. Will a stone float on water?
2. Are there fish in the sea?
3. Does one pound weigh more than two?
4. Can you use a hammer to pound a nail?

Command: "Hold up this many fingers" (Hold up 2 fingers)
"Now do the same thing with the other hand" (Do not demonstrate)
OR "Add one more finger" (If patient unable to move both arms)

→ > 1 Error → **CAM-ICU positive DELIRIUM Present**

→ 0-1 Error → **CAM-ICU negative NO DELIRIUM**

Copyright © 2002, E. Wesley Ely, MD, MPH and Vanderbilt University, all rights reserved

Neurological Assessment

Chapter 11

National Institute of Health Stroke Scale (NIHSS) Assessment

- The NIHSS is a tool used by physicians and nurses to objectively quantify the impairment caused by a stroke.
- The NIHSS is composed of 11 items, each of which scores a specific ability between 0 and 4.
- For each item, a score of 0 typically indicates normal function in that specific ability, while a higher score is indicative of some level of impairment.
- The patient's score from each item is summed in order to calculate the total NIHSS score.
- The maximum possible score is 42, with the minimum score of 0.
- NIHSS recommends the assessment be completed as a baseline prior to treatment, at 2 hours post treatment, at 24 hours, at 7 to 10 days, and at 3 months post stroke.

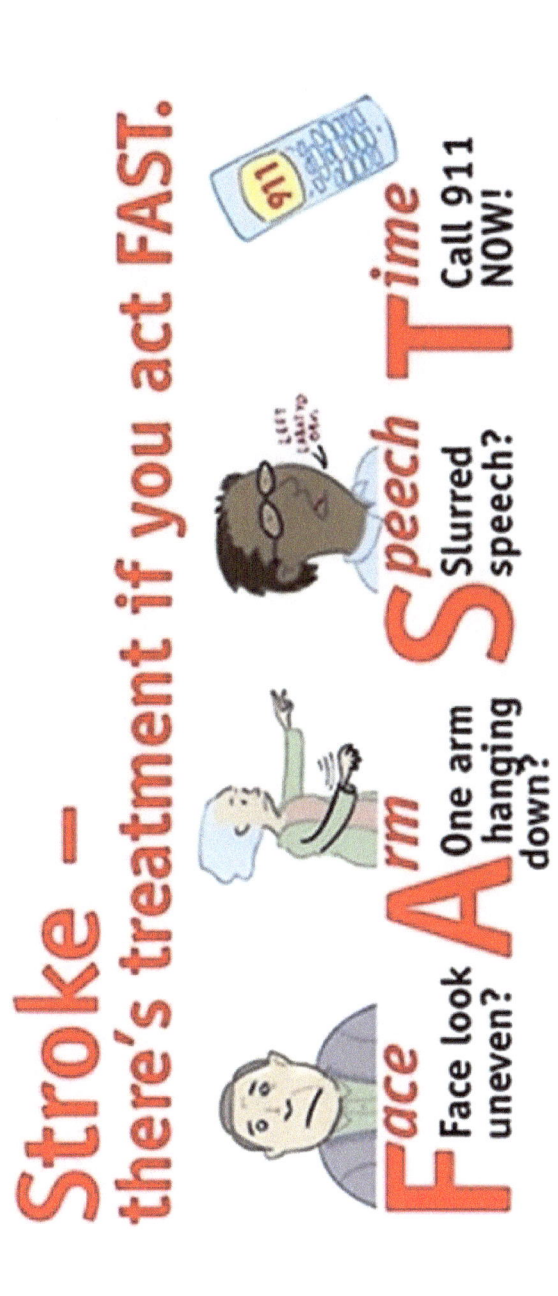

National Institutes of Health Stroke Scale

Score = 0   No stroke
Score = 1-4   Minor stroke

Score = 5-15 Moderate stroke
Score = 15-20 Moderate to severe stroke
Score = 21-42 Severe stroke

National Institutes of Health Stroke Scale score

1a. Level of consciousness	0 = Alert; keenly responsive 1 = Not alert, but arousable by minor stimulation 2 = Not alert; requires repeated stimulation 3 = Unresponsive or responds only with reflex

1b. Level of consciousness questions:
  What is the month?
  What is your age?
	0 = Answers two questions correctly
	1 = Answers one question correctly
	2 = Answers neither question correctly

1c. Level of consciousness commands:
  Open and close your eyes.
  Grip and release your hand.
	0 = Performs both tasks correctly
	1 = Performs one task correctly
	2 = Performs neither task correctly

2. Best gaze	0 = Normal 1 = Partial gaze palsy 2 = Forced deviation
3. Visual	0 = No visual loss 1 = Partial hemianopia 2 = Complete hemianopia 3 = Bilateral hemianopia
4. Facial palsy	0 = Normal symmetric movements 1 = Minor paralysis 2 = Partial paralysis 3 = Complete paralysis of one or both sides

5. Motor arm
  5a. Left arm
  5b. Right arm
	0 = No drift
	1 = Drift
	2 = Some effort against gravity
	3 = No effort against gravity; limb falls
	4 = No movement

6. Motor leg
  6a. Left leg
  6b. Right leg
	0 = No drift
	1 = Drift
	2 = Some effort against gravity
	3 = No effort against gravity
	4 = No movement

7. Limb ataxia	0 = Absent 1 = Present in one limb 2 = Present in two limbs
8. Sensory	0 = Normal; no sensory loss 1 = Mild-to-moderate sensory loss 2 = Severe to total sensory loss
9. Best language	0 = No aphasia; normal 1 = Mild to moderate aphasia 2 = Severe aphasia 3 = Mute, global aphasia
10. Dysarthria	0 = Normal 1 = Mild to moderate dysarthria 2 = Severe dysarthria
11. Extinction and inattention	0 = No abnormality 1 = Visual, tactile, auditory, spatial, or personal inattention 2 = Profound hemi-inattention or extinction

Total score = 0–42.

Chapter 12
Neurological Patient Case Studies

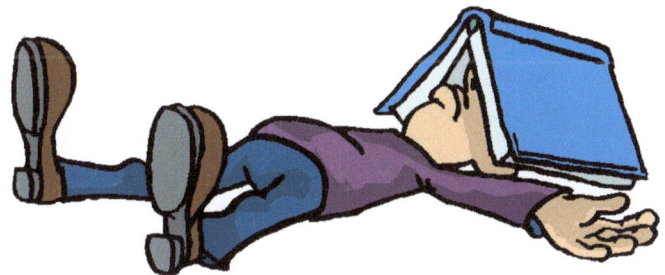

Please read each question and attempt to answer. Verify your thinking with the rationale.

1. A patient with head trauma develops a urine output of 300 ml/hour, dry skin, and dry mucous membranes. Which of the following nursing interventions is the most appropriate to perform initially?
    a. Evaluate urine specific gravity
    b. Anticipate treatment for renal failure
    c. Provide emollients to the skin to prevent breakdown
    d. Slow down the IV fluids and notify the physician

A. RATIONALE: A high urine output of 300 ml/hour may indicate diabetes insipidus, which is a failure of the pituitary gland to produce anti-diuretic hormone. This may occur with increased intracranial pressure and head trauma. The nurse should evaluate for low urine specific gravity, increased serum osmolarity, and dehydration. There is no evidence that the patient is experiencing renal failure. Providing emollients to prevent skin breakdown is important, but does not need to be performed immediately. Slowing the rate of IV fluid would contribute to dehydration when polyuria is present.

2. When evaluating an Arterial Blood Gas (ABG) from a patient with a subdural hematoma, the nurse notes the PaCO2 is 30 mm Hg. Which of the following responses best describes this result?
    a. Appropriate; lowering carbon dioxide (CO2) reduces intracranial pressure (ICP).
    b. Emergent; the patient is poorly oxygenated.
    c. Normal
    d. Significant; the patient has alveolar hypoventilation.

A. RATIONALE: A normal PaCO2 value is 35 to 45 mm Hg. CO2 has vasodilating properties which increase Intracranial Pressure (ICP). Therefore, lowering the PaCO2 to 30 mm Hg via hyperventilation will lower ICP and decrease the risk of further bleeding. Oxygenation is evaluated through PaO2 and oxygen saturation. Alveolar hypoventilation would cause an increase in PaCO2.

3. A patient with a complete C6 spinal injury would most likely have which of the following symptoms?
    a. Aphasia
    b. Hemiparesis
    c. Paraplegia
    d. Tetraplegia

D. RATIONALE: Tetraplegia occurs as a result of cervical spine injuries. Paraplegia occurs as a result of injury to the thoracic cord and below. Hemiparesis is one-sided paralysis that occurs as a result of an incomplete spinal cord injury. Aphasia usually occurs as the result of a stroke.

4. While in the Emergency Department, a patient with C8 tetraplegia develops a blood pressure of 80/40, pulse of 48, and respiratory rate of 18. The nurse suspects which of the following conditions?
    a. Autonomic dysreflexia
    b. Hemorrhagic shock
    c. Neurogenic shock
    d. Pulmonary embolism

C. RATIONALE: Symptoms of neurogenic shock include hypotension, bradycardia, and warm, dry skin due to the loss of adrenergic stimulation below the level of the lesion. Hypertension, bradycardia, flushing, and sweating of the skin are seen with autonomic dysreflexia. Hemorrhagic shock presents with anxiety, tachycardia, and hypotension. This would not be suspected without an injury. Pulmonary embolism presents with chest pain, hypotension, hypoxemia, tachycardia, and hemoptysis. Due to prolonged immobility, pulmonary embolism may develop as a later complication of spinal cord injury.

5. A 22-year-old patient with quadriplegia is apprehensive and flushed, with a blood pressure of 210/100 and a heart rate of 50 bpm. Which of the following nursing interventions should be done first?
   a. Place the patient flat in bed
   b. Assess patency of the indwelling urinary catheter
   c. Give one sublingual (SL) nitroglycerin tablet
   d. Raise the head of the bed (HOB) immediately to 90 degrees

D then B. RATIONALE: Anxiety, flushing above the level of the lesion, piloerection, hypertension, and bradycardia are symptoms of autonomic dysreflexia, typically caused by noxious stimuli such as a full bladder, fecal impaction, or decubitus ulcer. Putting the patient flat will cause the blood pressure to increase even more. The indwelling urinary catheter should be assessed immediately after the head of the bed (HOB) is raised. Nitroglycerin is given to reduce chest pain and reduce preload. It is not used for hypertension or dysreflexia.

6. A patient is admitted to the ER for head trauma and diagnosed with an epidural hematoma. The underlying cause of epidural hematoma is usually related to which of the following conditions?
    a. Laceration of the middle meningeal artery
    b. Rupture of the carotid artery
    c. Thromboembolism from a carotid artery
    d. Venous bleeding from the arachnoid space

A. RATIONALE: Epidural hematoma or extradural hematoma is usually caused by laceration of the middle meningeal artery. A ruptured carotid artery (carotid blowout syndrome) tends to occur in patients with neck cancer or post neck radiation therapy. A ruptured carotid artery will not result in an epidural bleed. Thromboembolism that travels to the brain from the carotid artery can cause an embolic stroke. Venous bleeding from the arachnoid space is usually observed with subdural hematoma.

7. Which of the following conditions indicates that spinal shock is resolving in a patient with C7 quadriplegia?
    a. Absence of pain sensation in chest
    b. Spasticity
    c. Spontaneous respirations
    d. Urinary continence

B. RATIONALE: Spinal or neurogenic shock is characterized by hypotension, bradycardia, dry skin, flaccid paralysis, or the absence of reflexes below the level of injury (C7). Spasticity, the return of reflexes, is a sign of resolving shock. The absence of pain sensation in the chest does not apply to spinal shock. Respiratory difficulties will only occur if the level of injury is at C4 or above. C7 quadriplegia is characterized by a permanent loss of bladder control.

8. A patient with a T1 spinal cord injury arrives at the Emergency Department with a BP of 82/40, pulse of 34, dry skin, and flaccid paralysis of the lower extremities. Which of the following conditions would most likely be suspected?
   a. Autonomic dysreflexia
   b. Hypervolemia
   c. Neurogenic shock
   d. Sepsis

C. RATIONALE: Loss of sympathetic control and unopposed vagal stimulation below the level of injury typically cause hypotension, bradycardia, pallor, flaccid paralysis, and warm, dry skin in the patient with neurogenic shock. Hypervolemia is indicated by rapid and bounding pulse and edema. Autonomic dysreflexia occurs after neurogenic shock abates. Signs of sepsis would include elevated temperature, increased heart rate, and increased respiratory rate.

9. The nurse is discussing the purpose of an electroencephalogram (EEG) with the family of a patient who has massive cerebral hemorrhage and loss of consciousness. It would be most accurate for the nurse to tell family members that the test measures which of the following conditions?
   a. Extent of intracranial bleeding
   b. Sites of brain injury
   c. Activity of the brain
   d. Percent of functional brain tissue

C. RATIONALE: An EEG measures the electrical activity of the brain. Extent of intracranial bleeding and location of the injury site would be determined by CT or MRI. Percent of functional brain tissue would be determined by a series of tests.

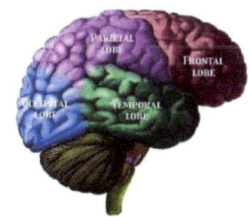

10. A patient arrives at the ER after slipping on a patch of ice and hitting her head. A CT scan of the head shows a collection of blood between the skull and dura mater. Which type of head injury does this finding suggest?
    a. Subdural hematoma
    b. Subarachnoid hemorrhage
    c. Epidural hematoma
    d. Contusion

C. RATIONALE: An epidural hematoma occurs when arterial blood collects between the skull and the dura mater. In a subdural hematoma, venous blood collects between the dura mater and the arachnoid mater. In a subarachnoid hemorrhage, blood collects between the pia mater and arachnoid membrane, usually as a result of a ruptured aneurysm. A contusion is a bruise on the brain's surface.

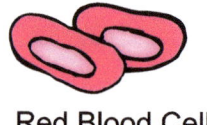

Red Blood Cell

11. The nurse is caring for a patient with a T5 complete spinal cord injury. Upon assessment, the nurse notes flushed skin, diaphoresis above T5, and a blood pressure of 162/96. The patient reports a severe, pounding headache. Which of the following nursing interventions would be appropriate for this patient? Select all that apply.
    a. Elevate the head of bed (HOB) to 90 degrees
    b. Loosen constrictive clothing
    c. Use a fan to reduce diaphoresis
    d. Assess for bladder distention and bowel impaction

A. B. & D. RATIONALE: The patient has signs and symptoms of autonomic dysreflexia. The potentially life-threatening condition is caused by an uninhibited response from the sympathetic nervous system resulting from a lack of control over the autonomic nervous system. The nurse should immediately elevate the head of the bed (HOB) to 90 degrees to reduce blood pressure while placing the extremities in a dependent position to decrease venous return to the heart.

Because tactile stimuli can trigger autonomic dysreflexia, any constrictive clothing should be loosened. The nurse should also assess for bladder distention and bowel impaction, which may trigger autonomic dysreflexia. Elevated blood pressure is the most life-threatening complication of autonomic dysreflexia because it can cause stroke, MI, or seizures. If removing the triggering event does not reduce the patient's blood pressure, IV antihypertensives should be administered. A fan should not be used because cold drafts may actually trigger autonomic dysreflexia.

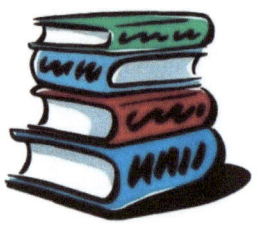

12. The patient with a head injury has been urinating copious amounts of dilute urine through their Foley catheter. The patient's urine output for the previous 12-hour shift was 3000 ml. The nurse implements a new physician order to administer:
    a. Desmopressin (DDAVP)
    b. Dexamethasone (Decadron)
    c. Ethacrynic acid (Edecrin)
    d. Mannitol (Osmitrol)

A. RATIONALE: Desmopressin (DDAVP). A complication of a head injury is diabetes insipidus, which can occur when there is insult to the hypothalamus, the antidiuretic storage vesicles, or the posterior pituitary gland. Urine output that exceeds the normal urine output of 800 to 2000 mL per day generally requires treatment with desmopressin. Dexamethasone, a steroid, is administered to treat cerebral edema. Ethacrynic acid and Mannitol are diuretics, which would be contraindicated.

13. The nurse is caring for a patient in the Emergency Department following a head injury. The patient momentarily lost consciousness at the time of the injury and then regained it. The patient now has lost consciousness again. The nurse takes quick action, knowing this is compatible with:
    a. Skull fracture
    b. Concussion
    c. Subdural hematoma
    d. Epidural hematoma

D. RATIONALE: The neurological changes from an epidural hematoma begin with a loss of consciousness as arterial blood collects in the epidural space and exerts pressure. The patient regains consciousness as the cerebral spinal fluid is reabsorbed rapidly to compensate for the rising intracranial pressure. As the compensatory mechanisms fail, even small amounts of additional blood can cause the intracranial pressure to rise rapidly, and the patient's neurological status deteriorates quickly.

14. A patient has been pronounced brain dead. Which findings would the nurse assess? Check all that apply.
   a. Decerebrate posturing
   b. Dilated non-reactive pupils
   c. Deep tendon reflexes
   d. Absent corneal reflex

B. C. & D. RATIONALE: A patient who is brain dead typically demonstrates non-reactive dilated pupils and non-reactive or absent corneal and gag reflexes. The patient may still have spinal reflexes such as deep tendon and Babinski reflexes in brain death. Decerebrate or decorticate posturing would not be observed when the patient is brain dead.

Sedation and Epidural Anesthesia Questions

15. List the most appropriate actions when a patient has a severe adverse reaction to opioid medication with respiratory rate of 7 and oxygen saturation of 86%.

    ANSWER: Stimulate, open airway, administer O2, notify the physician, and anticipate administration of reversal agents.

16. The nurse administers Naloxone to the patient with respiratory depression secondary to morphine. Initially the patient has a positive response, with increased respiratory effort, but after 45 minutes, the patient goes back to sleep and their respiratory rate decreases to 10 per minute. Which of the following explains what the nurse is observing?

    ANSWER: Naloxone has a shorter duration of action than morphine.

17. Define the criteria for moderate sedation / analgesia.

   ANSWER: Patient is sedated but able to follow commands, may require oxygen to maintain saturations greater than 92%, and is able to protect airway.

18. Monitoring and documentation of the patient's sedation score will continue until?

   ANSWER: The sedation score matches or exceeds their pre anesthesia or pre procedural score.

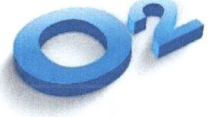

19. If your patient is receiving an anesthetic epidural agent, your assessments are to include. Select all that apply:
    a. Symptoms of postural hypotension.
    b. Head of the bed (HOB) at 30 degrees.
    c. Dermatome levels to assess sensory sensation.
    d. Vital signs, pain and sedation / level of consciousness (LOC) checks every 15 minutes for 1 hour, then every hour for 24 hours, then every 4 hours for the duration.

    ANSWER: All of the above

20. In the patient receiving epidural anesthesia, when motor and sensory functions begin to show impairment, what should the nurse suspect as the cause?
    a. Inadequate analgesia.
    b. Catheter migration.
    c. Residual anesthesia from surgery.
    d. Spinal cord damage during insertion of epidural catheter.

    ANSWER: Catheter migration.

21. All of the following are important considerations in ambulation of the patient with a Continuous Epidural Infusion containing Marcaine. Which would be the MOST important?
    a. Check motor sensation every time before the patient ambulates.
    b. Obtain an activity order from the anesthesiologist / MD.
    c. Allow the patient to ambulate independently if no problems have occurred previously.
    d. Upon completion of ambulation, recheck insertion site and security of dressing.

ANSWER: Check motor sensation every time before the patient ambulates.

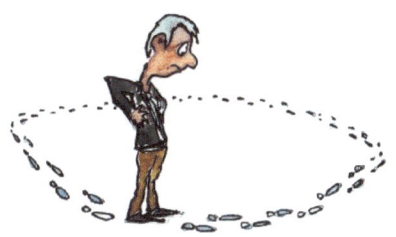

In Summary

This book is intended to help nurses effectively monitor patients for neurological changes by performing thorough neurological assessments.

The key to successful delivery of nursing care for neurological patients involves excellent assessment skills, attention to detail, and close communication of findings with the Neurologist, Neurosurgeon, Nurse Practitioner and Physician's Assistant.

Accurate neurological assessments are the basis for proper implementation of medical and nursing interventions in accordance with the patient's overall plan of care.

Notes: